Why Medicine?
And 500 Other Questions for the Medical School and Residency Interviews

Also by Sujay Kansagra

Everything I Learned in Medical School: Besides All the Book Stuff

Available from Amazon and other retailers!

Why Medicine?

And 500 Other Questions for the Medical School and Residency Interviews

By

Sujay M. Kansagra, MD

ISBN-13: 978-1479286348
ISBN-10: 1479286346

For the students all over the
world that know me as
Dr. K.

Contents

Why Medicine?

Preface

I vividly remember the interview process for medical school and residency. The process was long, arduous and expensive. It required hours of pasting a smile on my face and feeling as if someone was watching my every move. But the process was also a chance to meet others that were in my shoes, a chance to travel, and a chance to connect. This was my opportunity to shine and show these institutions the true person behind the application. With each passing interview, I became more comfortable and confident. The reason was simple… I felt prepared!

The process of applying to medical school and residency can be challenging. However, with the right preparation, it can also be an enjoyable and rewarding experience. The purpose of this book is to help you with this preparation. Good luck!

Chapter 1

How to Use this Book

The book's layout is simple. In the following pages you will find question after question. These are some of the most common questions that I encountered as an interviewee and asked as an interviewer. Notes and thoughts can be written in the space provided after each question. You should not write out entire answers! The trick to interviewing is being prepared with answers but not sounding rehearsed. This can be difficult. The best strategy is to develop some thoughts for each question but not memorize entire answers.

You will undoubtedly come across many questions that are not covered here. However, most questions along the interview trail become repetitive and can be anticipated. I've put these questions in this book.

Please realize that there are no answers in this book! The reason is simple: The answers should come from you. You should not simply regurgitate responses that you believe people want to hear. The entire purpose of the interview is for institutions to get to know you and determine if you are a good match for their program. They should be hearing your thoughts, not someone else's. Where appropriate, I have offered guidance on how to frame your answer. The actual answers should come from you.

Chapter 2
Interviewing Tips

Tip 1: Know your application

You will quickly discover that the majority of questions will be about your application. This works in your favor since you should know your application better than anyone else. Always keep a copy of the application with you and review it the night before your interview. Recall the type of work you did for each extracurricular activity. This is especially true for research. Never be caught saying, "I only cleaned the test tubes." Even if you just did manual labor, you should know the type of research the laboratory performed and their goals. Not knowing the details behind your activities is a major red flag and tells the interviewer that you participated superficially just to write it on your resume.

Tip 2: Know the location

I made it a habit to drive to the hospital the night before my interview so I knew exactly where I was going. Knowing the directions takes one stress away from what will already be a stressful day. Never trust Google Maps or your GPS. See it for yourself!

Tip 3: Time should be on your side

Nothing gets the interview day off to a worse start than running late. It creates stress for you, and if you do show up late, hurts your chances of acceptance. Instead, plan to get there 30 minutes earlier than scheduled. If you are there early, walk around or read over your application. Time should be your friend during the interview process.

Tip 4: Dress the part

The interview trail is not the place to experiment with the latest in fashion. Stick with the convention. For females, a suit is the norm with the skirt suit being the most common. A pant suit is perfectly acceptable. If you go with a skirt, make sure it is the appropriate length (to the knees). For men, a suit is a must. The colors for males and females are similar – stick with navy blue, black or grey. Avoid excessive perfume and cologne. They should remember you for what you said and not how you smelled.

Tip 5: Keep talking

The key to a successful interview is staying loose. I forced myself to make conversation with my fellow interviewees and talked about neutral topics that had nothing to do with the interview process. This was a great way to stay relaxed. Sitting in a corner by yourself and thinking about the upcoming interview may have the opposite effect.

Tip 6: Be honest

You have probably heard this advice countless times. The best way to ruin your chances of being offered a spot in a program is to lie. In addition, nothing gets you more nervous during an interview than stretching the truth. Not to mention that you are about to embark on a career path where your integrity and character mean everything. Stick with the truth.

THE
QUESTIONS

Chapter 3

Opening Questions

1. Tell me about yourself.

2. Where are you from?

3. Do you know anyone in this area?

4. What got you interested in our institution?

5. Where else are you applying? Have you already interviewed at these places?

6. What do you know about our school?

7. What have you seen so far?

It always impressed me as an interviewer when candidates remembered what they had seen on the tour and the interviewers they had already met. It showed me that they were interested.

8. Can you summarize your application for me?

Be succinct. You don't have to mention all of your accomplishments. You should never talk for more than one minute at a time. Therefore, hit the highlights and then give the interviewer the opportunity to ask more questions. The interview should feel like a conversation.

9. If you only had ten seconds to sell yourself, what would you say?

10. Why medicine?

This is a very common question. You can expect to hear this everywhere. Everyone says some variation of, "I like people and I like science". Try to be a little original. Personal stories are a plus.

Chapter 4
Your Application

1. Tell me about _____ (fill in the blank with one of your activities).

   Questions regarding activities from your application tend to be the most common questions. Anything from your application is fair game. Know your application well!

2. Which extracurricular activity are you most proud of?

3. Which activity took up most of your time?

4. Which activity was the most rewarding?

5. Which activity did you dislike and why?

6. What was your last volunteer activity?

7. How did you choose your extracurricular activities?

8. How did you have time to do so many activities?

   The hidden question here is, "Did you participate superficially to bulk up your application?" When this came up, I emphasized that I had diverse interests and that I managed my time well.

9. Why did you participate in so few activities?

   If this question comes up, emphasizing the extent of your involvement with your activities is important.

Interviewers should appreciate quality involvement over quantity.

10. Do you plan on staying involved with any of these extracurricular groups in the future?

11. Did you take on leadership roles in any of your activities?

    If you didn't have an official title in your activities, you can still mention specific projects or tasks in which you took the lead.

12. Which activities got you interested in medicine?

13. How have your experiences contributed toward preparing you for a career in medicine?

14. Did any of your activities involve direct patient contact?

15. Which activity do you truly feel made an impact on someone else?

16. Which activity had the biggest impact on you?

17. Tell me about some of your activities that had nothing to do with medicine.

18. Is there something from your application that you want to highlight?

19. How did you decide on your topic for the personal statement?

20. How well do you know the people that wrote your recommendation letters?

21. How did you choose the people that wrote your recommendation letters?

22. Have you had a chance to read any of your recommendations? If so, do you feel they are accurate?

23. What honor/award are you the most proud of? Why?

24. Which honor/award did you work the hardest to achieve?

25. Did you have any work experience while in college?

It is perfectly acceptable to not have any paid work experience. Most students do not.

26. Did you do any research while in college? If so, describe your research and its applications?

Many students do not have time or interest in research and that is okay. However it can be a big plus on your application. If you did research, remember that all scientific research endeavors have a human application. It is important to summarize the work of the lab in a way the interviewer can understand and then explain how this may benefit patients in the future.

27. What did you think about our application process?

Chapter 5

You

1. Have you always wanted to become a doctor?

2. How long ago did you decide you wanted to be a doctor?

3. What would you do if you couldn't go into medicine?

4. Have you ever had a job outside of the medical field?

5. What makes you, you?

6. Tell me something most people don't know about you.

7. What is a typical day for you?

8. Where were you born?

9. Describe your life growing up.

10. What is your first memory?

    The earliest memories are usually from around the age of three. Don't say you remember your birth.

11. Tell me about your family.

12. Is anyone in your family in medicine?

13. Which family member has influenced you the most?

14. What is the most important lesson your family has taught you?

15. Does your family support your decision to go into medicine?

16. Did anybody try to discourage you from a career in medicine?

17. Which qualities do you want to pass down to your kids?

18. Do you have any siblings? What are they like?

19. Who are your mentors?

20. If I had three of your former mentors in a room and asked them about you, what would they say?

21. What would your mentors say about you that you would say is not true?

    Try to emphasize something positive here. For example, your mentors would say you are "all work and no play", which you could say is not true.

22. Who has helped you the most in getting you to where you are today?

23. Who do you confide in?

24. Did anyone guide you toward a career in medicine?

25. So are you going into medicine for those other people or for yourself?

The point here is that you should choose medicine for yourself and not because your parents or siblings told you to. Important to emphasize that although people may have encouraged you toward a medical career, the ultimate decision was your own.

26. Who impresses you the most and why?

27. Do you consider yourself to be successful?

It is always good to take the confident yet humble route. Emphasizing you are proud of your accomplishments but stating you still have many

unmet goals usually does the trick.

28. Who depends on you?

29. If you have a personal problem, who do you go to for advice?

30. Who is the smartest person you know?

31. Who are you most proud of?

32. Who is your hero? Why?

33. What drives you?

34. What amazes you?

35. What are you passionate about?

36. What are your priorities in life?

37. What is your greatest skill?

38. What are your strengths?

39. What are your weaknesses?

Again, your answer should be something that can be seen as a positive. I would often say I have a hard time delegating because I like taking ownership of tasks. Another example would be that you have a hard time saying "no" and take too much onto your plate. People in medicine can usually relate to both of these "weaknesses".

40. What is your greatest fault?

41. If you were forced to change one thing about yourself, what would it be?

42. How do you handle failure?

43. What is your greatest achievement?

44. What is one thing you would change about your past?

45. If you could go through college again, would you do anything differently?

46. What bothers you?

47. What frightens you?

48. What makes you angry?

49. Who irritates you the most and why? How do you deal with that person?

50. What makes you laugh?

51. Do you think there is a role for humor in medicine?

52. Do you have a sense of humor?

53. What makes you the happiest?

54. What was the happiest day of your life?

55. What was the worst day of your life?

56. What fascinates you?

57. How would your friends describe you?

58. How many close friends do you have?

59. Who is your best friend? Describe him/her.

60. Describe your personality.

61. If you could change something about your personality, what would it be?

62. If you could describe yourself in three words, what would they be?

63. If you could look into the future, what would your tombstone say?

64. Where do you see yourself in 5 years?

65. Where do you see yourself in 10 years?

66. Where do you see yourself in 25 years?

67. At what age do you want to retire?

68. If you had enough money to retire at 40, would you?

69. Where in the world would you like to settle?

70. If you had to move to a country other than your home country, where would you go? Why?

71. Where have you travelled?

72. Where is the most interesting place you have travelled and why?

73. What are your hobbies?

74. What is your favorite book?

75. Do you read any magazines or newspapers regularly?

76. What is your favorite movie?

77. Do you have a favorite quote?

78. What is your favorite color and why?

79. What type of music do you like?

80. Do you play any sports?

81. What is your most prized possession?

82. Tell me about a time you had to give up something you loved.

83. Do you feel you have had to sacrifice anything by choosing this career path?

84. Do you think there will be future sacrifices you will have to make in order to be a doctor? Are you prepared to make those sacrifices?

85. Have you ever quit at something you were doing? Why?

86. Tell me about a time you had to take a stand.

87. Tell me about a time you took on a leadership role.

88. What does it take to be a leader?

89. Tell me about how you handle conflict as a leader.

90. Tell me about a time you went above and beyond what was expected of you.

91. Have you ever helped someone when no one else would?

92. Is your life different from what you imagined it would be?

93. What is your philosophy...do you "live to work", or "work to live"?

94. As a doctor, do you think you will "bring work home with you"?

95. Are you a risk taker?

96. Are you a good listener?

97. Are you self-aware?

98. Are you proactive? Give me an example.

99. Are you dependable? Give me an example.

100. Are you trustworthy? Give me an example.

101. Are you honest? Give me an example.

102. Are you organized? Give me an example.

103. Are you punctual?

104. Can you multitask? Give me an example.

105. Are you confident?

106. What activity do you feel most confident doing?

107. How do you show confidence without being arrogant?

108. What keeps you focused?

109. What are your biggest distractions?

110. How do you handle fatigue and sleep deprivation?

111. How do you know when you are tired?

112. How do you prioritize your activities?

113. Are you good at time management?

114. How do you divide up your time between work and family/friends?

115. When faced with a choice, are you thoughtful and analytical or do you usually make up your mind quickly? Give an example.

They may watch how fast you respond to this question to get their real answer.

116. Give me an example of a time when you had to make a split second decision.

117. Do you have any plans for your summer?

118. How good are you with computers and technology?

119. What is the biggest lesson you have learned in your life?

120. What have you done recently that you will remember forever?

121. What worries you the most about the future?

122. What about medical school/residency scares you the most?

123. What about medical school/residency do you think will be the most fun?

124. How do you battle against procrastination?

125. What is your motto?

126. What is the best decision you've ever made?

127. What was your toughest decision in the last six months? What made it difficult?

128. The last time you did not know which decision to make, what did you do?

129. What process do you go through to make important decisions affecting your career?

130. What do you do more often, ask questions or answer them?

131. What is one thing that would prevent you from going to medical school /practicing medicine?

132. Tell me about something you have not achieved yet.

133. How do you intend to achieve it?

134. Gandhi said, "Be the change you want to see in the world". What change do you want to see in the world?

135. Are you exemplifying this change?

136. What is the best part about being you?

Chapter 6
Character

1. A life in medicine means a life of service to others. How have you shown your dedication to serving others?

2. If you want to help others, why not go into social work instead?

3. What does it mean to have good character?

4. Tell me about a moral dilemma you've had and how you handled it.

5. What would you do if you saw your friend cheating on a test?

6. Have you ever done something you later regretted? How did you handle it?

7. What do you regret the most in your life?

8. Have you ever had to lie?

9. Is lying sometimes okay?

10. What is the biggest lie you've told someone?

11. Is asking for help a weakness or strength?

12. What is the Hippocratic Oath?

13. What does, "First, do no harm" mean to you?

14. What would you do if you found a large sum of money in the street?

15. A Jehovah's witness refuses a blood transfusion that you feel will be life saving. What do you do?

In these situations, the typical course of action is to obey the patient's wishes if you feel they are mentally capable of making such decisions and optimize their care as best as possible. Your goal as a doctor is ensuring they understand the risks and benefits of each course of action. If you feel the patient's thinking is compromised in any way, you have to treat based on standard of care with the involvement of close family members. Hospitals typically have ethics committees that also get involved with these types of cases.

16. What would you do if a patient has a curable cancer but refuses treatment?

Same approach applies here as prior question.

17. Your family member asks for a prescription for a medication. What would you do?

The right answer is that you would not prescribe anything for family members. It is seen as unethical to prescribe medications for you or for family members, not to mention it's unsafe.

18. What are your top three personal values?

19. Do you have a moral rule that you would never break?

20. Would you prefer to provide less effective treatment to more patients or more effective treatment to fewer patients?

21. If you had the choice of giving a transplant to a successful elderly member of the community or a 20-year-old drug addict, who would you choose?

22. What does "empathy" mean to you?

23. How do you differentiate empathy from sympathy?

24. Do you feel that most doctors understand what their patients are going through?

Chapter 7
Patient Care

1. Have you had a chance to work in a hospital?

2. Have you interacted with patients? Tell me about your experience.

3. Do you think patients will find you personable?

4. What characteristics would you want in your doctor?

5. Which of your characteristics will make you a good doctor?

6. How will you know if you are being a good doctor?

7. How would you give someone bad news?

8. Let's pretend you just made a mistake and accidentally got a chest X-ray on the wrong patient. What would you do next?

9. Let's say you made a mistake that led to a patient dying. What would you do next? How would you handle that?

10. A patient waited two hours for you and is upset. What would you say to calm the patient down?

11. Is it more important to see all of your patients on time or to give each patient as much time as they want?

12. How do you think patients feel when you attribute their medical problems to their weight? How do you approach this discussion so that you don't offend them?

13. Have you ever been a patient? If so, tell me about your experience.

14. Have you ever had to stay overnight in a hospital?

15. What does patient-centered care mean to you?

16. Patients have access to medical information through the internet. Is this a good thing or a bad thing?

17. How would you tell a patient that he/she is wrong about something?

18. How would you deal with a patient that won't follow your advice or is noncompliant with medications?

19. What can physicians do to improve patient compliance from the start?

20. How can we improve compliance amongst physicians for important habits like hand washing?

21. How do you think you would handle the death of one of your patients?

22. What do you think you can contribute to the field of medicine?

23. What do you dislike about medicine?

24. Should doctors follow the same advice they give to their patients, such as eating healthy, exercising and not smoking?

25. What quality is most important in a doctor?

26. Which is more important, an intelligent doctor or a compassionate doctor?

27. Can compassion be taught?

28. Do you need compassion to be a successful doctor?

29. Do you think it is possible to become too emotionally attached to patients? Could it affect decision making?

30. Which are more important, communication skills or clinical skills?

31. It seems that students and residents often have a hard time speaking up when they

feel that their attendings are making a mistake. Why do you think that is?

32. Which is more important, an intelligent doctor or one with common sense?

33. What do you think about herbal remedies?

34. If a patient opted to use only herbal medicines for cancer, what would you tell them?

35. What do you think about acupuncture?

36. How do you stay up to date with the latest research in medicine?

37. What is the most important research we as a field should be doing in medicine?

38. What medical problem do you think will be cured next?

39. What medical problem do you think will never have a cure?

40. What would you say if a patient refused to be seen by you because of your gender or race?

41. What would you say if a patient tells you that you are too young to be a doctor?

42. How would you work to promote good health amongst society other than just seeing patients in clinic?

43. What social issues do you think you could address as a physician in your community?

44. Should medical education focus more on treating disease or preventing disease?

45. Doctors have to treat people from many different backgrounds. Have you been exposed to diversity in your life?

46. Do you speak any other languages?

47. What in your life has allowed you to become open-minded?

48. Is there any type of person that you would refuse to work with?

49. What can your future patients expect from you?

50. What should we expect from you?

51. What do you expect from us?

52. What expectations do you have of your future patients?

53. What does it mean to be "jaded" in medicine?

54. Why do you think so many doctors become jaded?

55. Why do doctors wear white coats if they carry microbes that can be harmful to patients? Should we get rid of white coats?

56. How do you think the role of doctors will change in 25 years? 100 years? 1000 years?

57. What will be the future role of doctors if computers are being developed that can develop sophisticated differentials based just on symptoms?

58. What medical procedures have you seen?

59. How do you handle seeing blood and gore? Do they bother you?

Chapter 8

Academics

1. What is your favorite subject?

2. What is your least favorite subject?

3. What was your favorite class in college?

4. What was your least favorite class in college?

5. Did you consider high school challenging?

6. Did you consider college challenging?

7. Which class was the most challenging?

8. Which class was the most entertaining?

9. Which class do you recommend all students take during undergrad?

10. Tell me about a class you did really well in.

11. Tell me about a class you did poorly in. Why did you do poorly?

12. How big was your high school/college?

13. What was your class rank in high school?

14. Do you think your college GPA reflects your abilities?

15. Do you think your SAT/MCAT/ USMLE score reflects your abilities?

16. Tell me about your favorite teacher.

17. What makes a good teacher?

18. Are you a good teacher?

19. How do you study for tests?

20. How many hours do you typically study each day?

21. What type of environment do you learn best in?

22. Do you like to study independently or with a group?

23. Are you a good test taker?

24. Are there any poor grades you'd like to take some time to explain?

25. Doctors are students for life. Are you comfortable with this?

26. What do you do when you run across something you don't know the answer to?

27. What resources do you use when you don't know something?

28. Do you think it's more important to know everything or know where to find the answers?

29. A patient asks you a question that you don't know the answer to. What do you say?

30. Do you think medical training takes too long?

Chapter 9

Teamwork

1. Do you work well with others?

2. What can your colleagues expect from you?

3. Are you more of a leader or a follower?

4. How would you describe your leadership style?

5. Tell me about a time you had a conflict with someone. How did you resolve it?

6. Are you reliable? Give me an example.

7. Are you comfortable delegating work?

8. Would you have a hard time handing off work to others at the end of a shift?

9. Do you like to work independently or as a team?

   The emphasis in all of medicine is on teamwork. So saying you are a loner probably won't fly well.

   .

10. How do you tell a peer that he/she is wrong about something?

11. How do you tell a superior that he/she is wrong about something?

12. When was the last time someone told you that you were wrong about something?

13. What's the best way to give feedback?

   Good feedback typically involves telling someone what they are doing right in addition to what they need to improve upon. Some people use the "feedback sandwich" in which they say something positive, then discuss an area that needs improvement, and conclude with another positive.

14. How do you like to receive feedback?

15. Do you think doctors have big egos? Why or why not?

16. Do you work best if someone sets expectations for you or if you establish goals independently?

   Self-motivation is a good trait to have in medicine.

17. What qualities do you look for in your colleagues?

Chapter 10
"If" Questions

1. If money wasn't an issue, which job would you choose and why?

   You should obviously still pick medicine; otherwise they will assume you are just doing this for the money.

2. If you could have dinner with anyone, living or deceased, who would you pick and why?

3. If you could have dinner with three people, living or deceased, who would they be and why?

4. If you were stranded on a deserted island, which three items would you take with you?

5. If you could cure one disease, which one would it be?

6. If you could relive any moment in your life, which moment would you choose?

7. If you had $1,000,000 to give away, who would you give it to?

8. If you could tell me one thing about yourself, what would it be?

9. If I had only one spot left for an applicant, what would you say to convince me I should accept you?

10. If you could live in any time period in history (past, present, or future), which period would you live in?

11. If you were an animal, which animal would you be?

12. If you were a kitchen appliance, which one would you be and why?

13. If you were a road sign, what would you say?

14. If you could have any superpower, which one would it be?

15. If you were given one year off to travel, where would you go?

16. If the world was going to end tomorrow, what would you do today?

17. If the world was going to end tomorrow, what would you do today besides spend time with family?

18. If you could send a message to the entire world, what would it say?

19. If you could add one thing to everyone's drinking water, what would it be?

20. If you came across a stranger in the road needing CPR, would you perform mouth-to-mouth?

Recently there has been more emphasis placed on the importance of the chest compression portion of CPR. The choice of doing mouth-to-mouth on a stranger is an individual decision, and it is perfectly acceptable to say you would not perform mouth-to-mouth due to possible exposure to body fluids that may put your health at risk.

21. If you were a teacher, what would you be teaching?

22. If you could ask anyone (dead or alive) one question, who would you ask and what would you ask them?

23. If you could instantly learn one language fluently, which language would you choose?

24. If Hollywood made a movie about you, who would you want to play the lead role?

25. If you could save one object in your house from a fire, what would you save?

26. If you had one day to do anything besides medicine, what would you do? What if you had one year?

27. If you found a magic lamp, what would your three wishes be?

28. If you had to lose one of your senses, which one would you pick?

29. If you ran the country, what is one piece of legislation you would propose?

30. If you were me, what question would you ask candidates?

Chapter 11

Healthcare Policy/Current Events

1. Tell me about the latest healthcare events in our country.

2. Do you think we have a good healthcare system?

3. What is your opinion on the status of our health care system as it stands?

4. How does the American system compare with the system in countries like Canada and England?

The main difference is that England and Canada have publicly funded healthcare whereas the US has a privatized system. That means in England and Canada, everyone contributes to the cost of healthcare through taxes. Access to the doctor is granted to everyone and the expenses are covered. In America, tax money does not support healthcare (with the exception of Medicare and Medicaid). Therefore, the average citizen has to pay for private insurance in order for medical expenses to be covered.

5. Which system is better?

The main advantage of nationalized healthcare is that everyone is covered. Opponents of nationalized healthcare say it creates a long waitlist and poor quality. There are plenty of other pros and cons of each system, but this should be all you need to know for an interview.

6. Why is healthcare so expensive?

   This question can have plenty of answers. Some common contributors to healthcare costs are excessive amounts of procedures and lab tests (perhaps to avoid a possible lawsuit), expensive equipment, and a population that is living longer and is sicker due to obesity.

7. Are doctors' salaries too high or too low?

8. If you could change one thing about the healthcare system, what would you change?

9. Are private, for-profit pharmaceutical companies a good thing or a bad thing for our healthcare system?

10. Should patients be allowed to purchase prescription drugs from Canada or Mexico?

11. Do you think it is okay for drug companies to advertise on television?

12. Is it okay for drug companies to provide free lunches for doctors?

13. Do you think it is beneficial for patients to have access to medical advice and information online?

14. What do you think about electronic medical records?

15. If an insurance company denies a patient a treatment you think they need, what would you do?

Physicians can appeal decisions and write to insurance companies. Always fight for your patient!

16. What do you think about stem cell research?

The overall sentiment amongst the medical community is that stem cell research is a promising area with the potential for great benefit to patient care.

17. Do you think that people should be allowed to not own health insurance if they wish?

18. Should physicians offer free care to those without insurance or does this just encourage people to not own health insurance?

19. Is it the government's right to put bans/limits on food and drinks in the interest of public health?

20. How much should the government be involved in healthcare?

Chapter 12

Questions Specific to the Medical School Interview

1. What do you like best about our school?

2. What are you looking for in a medical school?

3. What do you think is the goal of a medical school?

4. What do you have to offer our school?

5. What do you feel our school can offer you?

6. What do like about our curriculum?

7. Do you know what type of doctor you want to be?

8. Do you have any research interests?

9. Do you want to do research in your future career? If so, won't that take time away from patient care?

10. Do you see yourself living in this city for the next four years?

11. What other schools are you applying to?

12. What would you do if you are not accepted to medical school?

13. What do you think will be the most difficult part of medical school?

14. What would you do if a resident keeps contradicting you in front of the attending?

15. What would you do if the resident keeps contradicting you in front of the patient?

16. In what part of the medical school curriculum do you think you will excel?

17. In what part of the medical school curriculum do you think you will struggle?

18. What part of medical school are you most looking forward too?

19. How was your college experience?

20. How did you decide on your major?

21. Do you think college is necessary, or should students go straight from high school into medical school like they do in some other countries?

22. What do you think is the average day in the life of a physician?

23. Have you had the chance to work alongside a physician?

24. If you were accepted into multiple schools, how would you decide between them?

25. What advice would you give to a pre-med student who is just starting college?

26. Do you feel you are ready for the academic workload in medical school?

27. Do you feel you are ready for the responsibility of medical school?

28. Are you bothered by blood and gore?

29. Do you think medical school tuitions are too high?

30. Is there something about our school you do not like?

31. Do you think the admissions process to medical school is a fair process?

32. Are you interested in primary care or a specialty?

    It is okay not to know at this point in your education.

33. What specialty are you interested in?

34. What types of cases do you think someone in that specialty will see?

Chapter 13

Questions Specific to the Residency Interview

1. How did you decide on this field of medicine?

2. Tell me about your most interesting patient from medical school.

3. Tell me about your most difficult patient encounter from medical school.

4. How has your view of medicine changed after going through medical school?

5. What do you think about the new changes in work hours for interns and residents?

6. What are the advantages and disadvantages of limiting resident duty hours?

   The biggest advantage is having well rested residents who are less prone to making errors due to fatigue/sleepiness. Limiting work hours also puts residents at less risk of accidents when they drive home after long call shifts. Some disadvantages include having to constantly hand off patients to the next provider which can hurt patient care. You may also not get to see as many cases and thus learn less as a resident if your work hours are limited.

7. Do duty hours compromise patient care?

8. Are you a good communicator?

9. Explain to me how the heart works, and pretend I'm a random guy off the street.

10. What are the important parts to effective communication?

11. Residency is all about teamwork. Tell me about the last time you worked in a team?

12. What makes a good attending?

13. What is the role of a nurse?

14. What will be the future roles for physician extenders like nurse practitioners and physician assistants?

15. How do you deal with stress?

16. How do you deal with anxiety?

17. What do you think will be the most difficult part about residency?

18. In what aspect of residency do you think you will shine?

19. What part of residency are you most looking forward to?

20. What do you think will be the most challenging part of working in this specialty?

21. What other programs are you applying to?

22. What is the best way to teach medical students?

23. Have you had a chance to talk to our current residents? What have they told you?

24. If you suspected a fellow resident to be under the influence of drugs or alcohol while at work, what would you do?

    Patient care may be at risk in this situation. The right course of action would be to report the resident to the residency director.

25. If you felt a fellow resident had a problem with drugs or alcohol outside of work, what would you do?

    Again, if you feel patient care is being affected, you should go to the residency director.

26. How long does a good doctor spend talking to a patient during a clinic visit?

27. Have you ever felt rushed to see a patient? How did you handle it?

28. Did you ever feel uncomfortable examining a patient? How did you handle it?

29. Have you ever had to deal with an angry patient? How did you handle it?

30. Did you ever make a mistake in medical school that affected patient care?

31. How are you going to prevent malpractice suits during your career?

In addition to providing quality care, the best way to avoid lawsuits is to be upfront, honest, and build a strong patient-doctor relationship.

32. If I asked a patient you took care of during medical school about you, what would he/she say?

33. What patient stands out from your medical school experiences?

34. Pretend I'm a patient you are seeing in clinic for a simple viral upper respiratory infection. I am insisting I need antibiotics but you don't feel they are necessary. What would you tell me?

35. How much responsibility were you given on the wards in medical school?

36. What are the responsibilities of a doctor to a patient?

37. Did you get to perform procedures in medical school? If so, which ones?

38. How did your medical school prepare you to interview and examine patients?

39. Are you interested in academic medicine or private practice?

40. What are the advantages and disadvantages of a career in academic medicine?

41. What classes did you enjoy during medical school?

42. What classes did you not enjoy during medical school?

43. How were you graded in medical school?

44. Tell me about your curriculum during medical school. Did you enjoy it?

45. What would you change about your medical school's curriculum?

46. If you could do it over again, what would you change about your medical school experience?

47. If you could do it over again, would you choose the same medical school?

48. Would you tell your sibling/friend to pursue medicine now that you've been to medical school?

49. Did you consider medical school challenging?

50. How were you treated on the wards as a student? Will you treat students the same way or differently?

51. What did you do during medical school in your spare time?

52. What do you like to browse on the Internet?

53. Did you have time to read books apart from your textbooks?

54. Have you had to use an electronic medical record system? Did you like it?

55. Have you had to use a computerized order entry system? Did you find it easy to use?

56. Do you think an electronic medical record is better than a paper chart?

57. What are the components to a good patient history?

58. What advice would you give to someone just starting medical school?

59. Should residents get paid more?

60. How would you define "informed consent"?

61. How can you tell if you are getting through to a patient?

62. How do you counsel patients to make big lifestyle changes, such as with smoking, drugs, and healthy diet?

63. Should family members of the patient be present during a code?

64. When is it okay to restrain a patient?

65. Do you think the match is a fair process?

66. Will you be pursuing a fellowship?

67. If you had to choose a different specialty, which one would you choose?

Chapter 14

Questions for the Older Applicant

1. Why did you decide on a career in medicine so late?

2. How did you figure out that you wanted to be a doctor?

3. What did you do between college and the present?

4. Do you regret doing something else prior to applying to medical school?

5. How will you handle fatigue as an older student/resident?

6. Do you feel that being an older applicant is a disadvantage? How?

7. Do you feel that being an older applicant is an advantage? How?

8. What has your time out of school taught you?

9. Will you have enough time to pay back all of your loans? What is your plan?

Chapter 15

Questions You Probably Won't be Asked

This chapter title may sound silly, but there are many questions people warn you about during the interview, but in actuality, you are unlikely to hear them. This is because they are controversial and put applicants in an uncomfortable situation, which is not the purpose of the interview. Regardless, here are a few to think about.

1. What are your thoughts on abortion?

2. What are your thoughts on euthanasia?

3. Do you agree with Dr. Kevorkian?

4. Are you religious? Do you think religion should play a role in medicine?

5. Give me your opinion on the role of spirituality in healing.

6. What do you think about doing research on animals?

7. Have you ever had to deal with depression?

8. Have you ever had to deal with an anxiety disorder?

9. Should marijuana be legalized?

10. Do you have any problems with the ethics of animal cloning?

11. What do you think about the morning after pill?

12. Do you support a nationalized healthcare system?

13. Are you a Democrat or a Republican?

14. Is medicine a right or a privilege?

15. Are health insurance CEOs paid too much?

16. Teach me something.

17. *Insert any medical pimping question here.*

18. How smart are you?

19. Are you married?

20. Do you have kids? Do you plan on having children soon?

21. Do you really want to come here?

22. We think you are over qualified for a spot here. What do you think about that?

23. If I accepted you right now, would you say yes?

24. Where do we rank?

Chapter 16

Random Questions

1. Should sites like Facebook and Twitter be blocked in the workplace?

2. What do you love?

3. How do you measure success?

4. What is your dream job?

5. What is your nightmare job?

6. Have you ever been fired from a job? Why?

7. What is your favorite game?

8. What is your favorite organ in the human body?

9. How did you prepare for this interview?

10. When is the last time you tried something new?

11. Is stress a good or bad thing?

12. How do you feel about websites that rate physicians?

13. Would you rather be a worried genius or a carefree idiot?

14. Is there such a thing as perfect?

15. Why do you think we need sleep?

16. If the human lifespan were only 40 years, what would you do differently with your life?

Chapter 17

Special Situations

1. Why did you have to take your MCAT/USMLE exam more than once?

2. Explain why you did so poorly in this class.

3. Why didn't you choose to major in a science subject?

4. Why did you choose to major in a science subject?

5. As a foreign medical graduate, why are you interested in residency in this country? Will

you go back to your home country or stay here after you are done with training?

6. Tell me about your time in the military. Will you continue to work as a doctor in the military? How long do you plan to spend in the military?

7. You quit your last job. How do I know you won't quit the medical field?

8. As a person with a disability, do you think this would get in the way of patient care in any way? What challenges do you foresee facing?

9. Why have you decided to apply to the MD/PhD joint program?

10. Tell me about the disciplinary action that was taken against you.

11. Tell me about why you have a misdemeanor/felony on your record.

Chapter 18

Medical trivia/General Knowledge

1. Who was Hippocrates?

   Hippocrates was an ancient Greek physician who is referred to as the "Father of Western Medicine". The Hippocratic Oath was thought to have been written by him, although recent evidence shows that it may actually have been written after his death.

2. Who was Sir William Osler?

   Osler was a Canadian physician and is often referred to as the "Father of Modern Medicine". He was one of the founding professors at Johns

Hopkins Hospital and was the first to take medical students outside of the classroom for bedside clinical education.

3. What is the difference between allopathic and osteopathic programs?

Both programs involve four years of training and have fairly similar curriculums. Allopathic schools lead to an "MD" degree at their completion whereas osteopathic programs award "DO" degrees. Both degrees are legally and professionally equivalent. One main difference is that osteopathic schools put an emphasis on the holistic perspective with the belief that each part of the body is interconnected and that the patient must be treated as a whole. Another difference is that osteopathic programs give training called OMM (osteopathic manipulative medicine), which is a hands-on approach to fixing problems within

the musculoskeletal system.

4. What is the difference between Medicare
    and Medicaid?

    Both are publically funded programs established in

    1965 that provide health insurance. Medicare

    provides coverage to those 65 years of age and

    older (as well as for younger people with

    disabilities and for those with end stage renal

    disease). Medicaid provides insurance for those

    with low incomes and minimal financial resources.

5. How does an HMO work?

    HMOs (Health Maintenance Organizations) are

    health insurance providers that require physicians

    with whom they have contracts to provide medical

    care in agreement with the HMO's guidelines and

restrictions. This typically leads to less expensive

care since physicians are limited in their ability to

order tests/studies. Patients are limited in whom

they can see for medical care.

6. Name some of the best medical/scientific journals.

The New England Journal of Medicine, the Journal

of the American Medical Association (JAMA),

Science, Lancet and Nature are a few.

7. What is the longest bone in the human body?

The femur

8. What is the longest muscle in the human body?

The sartorius muscle, which runs from the pelvis to the tibia below the knee.

Chapter 19

Closing Questions

1. Do you have any questions for me?

   Always have something ready to ask your interviewers. Try not to ask the same question to each interviewer. It is always a bonus if you ask a question about some specific part that is original to their program. Some examples of questions are listed in the next chapter.

2. What else do you want to tell me?

3. What is the one thing that you definitely want me to share with the admission's committee?

4. Do you think I've gotten a good sense of who you are?

5. How do I rate as an interviewer?

6. Is there anything you have not gotten a chance to see that you would like to see at our institution?

Chapter 20
Questions You Can Ask

As mentioned in the prior chapter, each interview typically concludes with the interviewer asking you if you have any remaining questions. Here are a few examples of questions you could ask. You only need to ask one or two. The point is to get more information about some aspect of the program that interests you and also show your interest in their program.

FOR THE MEDICAL SCHOOL INTERVIEW

1. I was looking into the curriculum here and was wondering about _____.

2. How early do students get to interact with real patients?

3. Do students have time to do research during medical school?

4. What are the common concerns from students here, if any?

5. What parts of the program do students tend to enjoy the most?

6. What types of activities do students participate in outside of the hospital?

7. Do you enjoy living in this area?

8. Will we get a chance to meet other students?

9. When do students typically take their board exams?

10. Are there opportunities to do away rotations?

11. Is there a medical Spanish class offered here?

12. What type of patient population do you see in the hospital? Is it diverse?

FOR THE RESIDENCY INTERVIEW

1. How many residents go on to do fellowships from this program?

2. What percentage of residents in this program typically goes into academics versus private practice?

3. How many residents have joined the faculty at this hospital in the last few years?

4. Do residents have activities that they organize outside of the hospital?

5. Is there a group amongst the residents that organizes social activities for everyone?

6. What type of patient population do you see in the hospital? Is it diverse?

7. How often do residents attend their own continuity clinic?

8. Do you like the medical records system here? Is it an electronic medical record?

9. How long have you worked in this hospital?

10. How did you decide to come here?

CONTRIBUTE!

Do you have a question to add? Send your question to:
medschooladvice1@gmail.com
and it may be included in the next version.

Do you follow Dr. K (@medschooladvice) on Twitter?

Notes

Notes

Notes

Made in the USA
Lexington, KY
10 August 2015